THE 7-11 METHOD OF STUDY

Four Hours to Mastering
Your Exams for Academic
and Professional Success

Hin H. Leong

CPA, CA, CGA, ACA, FCCA, FCPA, CA (M), ACPA
BAccSc – Bachelor of Accounting Science, University of Calgary
MSc – Master of Science in Professional Accountancy, University of London

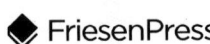 FriesenPress

Suite 300 - 990 Fort St
Victoria, BC, V8V 3K2
Canada

www.friesenpress.com

Copyright © 2019 by Hin H. Leong
First Edition — 2019

All rights reserved.

No part of this publication may be reproduced in any form, or by any means, electronic or mechanical, including photocopying, recording, or any information browsing, storage, or retrieval system, without permission in writing from FriesenPress.

ISBN
978-1-5255-3725-7 (Hardcover)
978-1-5255-3726-4 (Paperback)
978-1-5255-3727-1 (eBook)

1. STUDY AIDS

Distributed to the trade by The Ingram Book Company

Table of Contents

Preface vii

Chapter 1 1
Introduction

Chapter 2 5
First Week After The Course Registration

Chapter 3 11
First Month After The Course Starts

Chapter 4 15
Subsequent Months

Chapter 5 19
One Month Before The Final Exam

Chapter 6 23
Two Weeks Before The Final Exam

Chapter 7 27
The Day Before The Final Exam

Chapter 8 31
The Final Exam Day

Chapter 9 35
The Day After

Appendix A1. 38
Sample Planning Calendar
(After The Course Registration)

Appendix A2. 40
Sample Planning Calendar (Subsequent Month)

Appendix A3 42
Sample Planning Calendar
(One Month Before The Final Exam Day)

Appendix A4. 44
Blank Planning Calendar

Appendix B1. 46
Sample Daily Timetable

Appendix B2. 48
Blank Daily Timetable

About the Author 51

Preface

Hin H. Leong is a member in good standing of the Chartered Professional Accountants of Alberta and Canada (CPA, CA, CGA), an Associate Chartered Accountant of the Institute of Chartered Accountants in England and Wales (ACA), a Fellow of the Association of Chartered Certified Accountants of the United Kingdom (FCCA), a Fellow of the CPA Australia (FCPA), a Chartered Accountant of the Malaysian Institute of Accountants (CA (M)), and an ASEAN Chartered Professional Accountant (ACPA). He graduated from the University of London with a Master of Science in Professional Accountancy (MSc). He also has a Bachelor of Accounting Science degree from the Haskayne School of Business, University of Calgary, Alberta, Canada. In addition, he has a Diploma of Commerce (Financial Accounting) from Tunku Abdul Rahman University College in Kuala Lumpur, Malaysia.

Hin obtained the above credentials by sitting and passing challenging and often grueling exams from prestigious accountancy bodies around the world, including universities. Most of the exams were taken while working at a full time job and raising a family. He was often asked the secret of his success in passing exams, as many find it hard to get even one of the many credentials he has. He did it by faithfully following a disciplined and systematic approach that was perfected over time. Fortunately, it's easy to learn and emulate. Everyone can do it provided they put in the time and effort and have the will to succeed.

Hin is now ready to share his successful and proven method with you. This booklet is a compilation of years of experience of passing

THE 7-11 METHOD

exams, especially professional accountancy exams. If you are currently preparing for an exam, it will be a helpful guide and reminder of what you should do and how you should do it so that you will not only pass the dreaded exams but may even ace it.

Hin is also conducting a short training and seminar session to share his secret of success at locations and institutions of higher learning near you. He looks forward to meeting with you in person whenever the opportunity arises.

As you continue to study hard and prepare to write your exams, may the force be with you as you walk confidently into the exam hall and answer all the questions on the exam papers knowing that you are going to pass or ace it. Good luck!

Chapter 1
Introduction

Writing an exam can be a scary thought for many students, young and old, but it's what you sign up for when you decide to pursue a course of study. Exams are often the only measure of competency in a chosen field of study. Passing exams conducted by professional bodies is often more challenging than writing the academic exams administered by colleges and universities. Every year, thousands of students graduate with degrees from these institutions, but only a small percentage pursue professional study. Being a professional such as Chartered or Certified Public Accountant, you are almost guaranteed a successful career and a bright future. In this book, we will focus on how to prepare for and pass a professional accountancy exam, although the approach and method is universal in nature and can be applied to any exam you need to write.

Professional accountancy exams are often governed by a statutory recognized professional accountancy body of a country. For example, in Canada the body is now unified under the banner of CPA Canada, and a student successfully passing all the required CPA Canada exams, and completing the relevant work experience, is entitled to use the prestigious CPA designation. Other countries, such as Britain and Australia, have more than one statutory recognized professional accountancy body.

Accountants are the backbone of a country's economy. Many accountants run successful corporations around the world. They are usually gainfully employed regardless of the status of the country or the world's economy. We need more accountants, and accountants are ranked among the world's most trusted professionals.

To become a registered professional accountant, you must study and pass all the required exams and gain the relevant work experience. Once you decide to start the course, the journey can take many years. For some, it may even take more than a decade to complete their studies. Most people (like me) pursue professional study after they have graduated from college or university and started working. Some will get married and start a family along the journey (also like me).

The professional accountancy exams are not only very challenging but are a grueling test of stamina. The passing mark in a course used to be 50 per cent, but now a number of professional associations have raised it to 60 per cent with some as high as 75 per cent. A proper and disciplined approach to preparing for the exam is the key to success no matter how difficult the exam may be. Many people have done it already, and I am sure you can do it too.

Accounting courses are often divided into modules, and you have about ten to twelve weeks to complete the course. Assignments must be submitted on a weekly basis or at a pre-determined regular interval. Achieving a passing mark for each assignment is important because it qualifies you to write the final exam at the end of the course.

The exam is usually three to four hours long and often written after office hours starting from 6.00 p.m. or 7.00 p.m. on a weekday. Some exams may be conducted over several days or over the weekend. Because you will be writing in the evening or on the weekend, you need to ensure that you are both physically and mentally fit and well prepared for it. If you are already feeling exhausted at the end of a busy workday, you can imagine how much tougher it will be trying to write the exam a few hours later. That probably explains why the passing rate for professional exams is very low.

Once you take a seat in the exam hall, the pressure to get through it starts immediately. You will notice that students sitting around you are feeling as anxious as you are. This is normal. The tension begins to build as the proctor explains the exam procedures and distributes the papers. When the time to start finally arrives, there is no turning back. This is what you have been preparing for since you decided to take on the course; therefore, you need to concentrate on the task at hand, read the exam questions carefully, and answer each one to the best of your ability and knowledge.

If you have prepared well for this day, and the exam questions are what you expected, you will smile in your heart, knowing that you are going to make it or even ace it. On the other hand, if the exam questions are not what you anticipated but you studied all the course material provided, there is really nothing to panic about as all the other students will be feeling the same way. You just need to answer the questions to the best of your ability.

Time is a God-given treasure to all of us. It moves forward regardless of events, and it never turns back. Before you know it, the amount of time allocated for the exam is up and you are required to stop and hand in the answer sheets. If you have prepared well for the exam, you

THE 7-11 METHOD

will feel a sense of relief and accomplishment. Enjoy the few moments of triumphant victory. On the other hand, if you are unable to answer more than half of the questions, you may have to retake the exam, and this is not what you have prepared for.

Once the exam is submitted, there is really nothing you can do other than wait for your results. I cannot emphasize enough that it is extremely important for you to prepare well for the exam. You must put in all you have got from day one. Unfortunately, some will come to realize too late that failing an exam is no fun. It is demoralizing and a waste of your hard-earned money, not to mention the precious time spent studying over the last several months. Therefore, you must strive to pass the exam on your FIRST ATTEMPT.

Chapter 2
First Week After The Course Registration

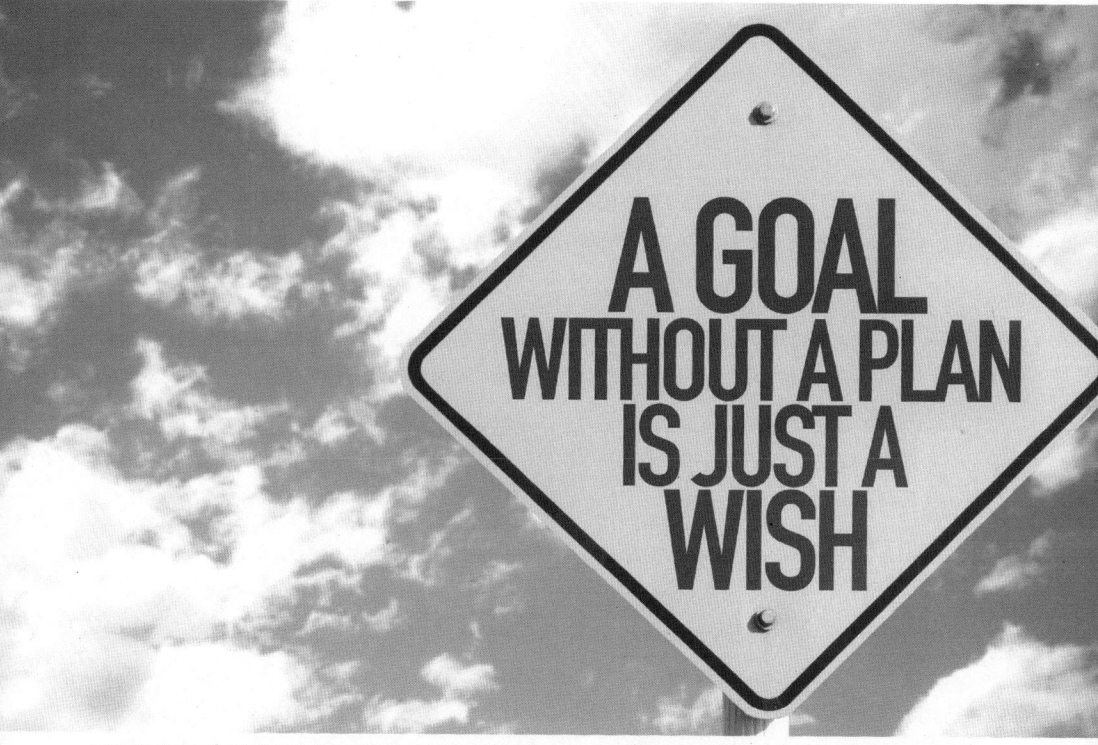

Most of us will feel motivated to start working on the course after signing up and paying the fees. We are embarking on a new "adventure." Since we have paid a lot of money for it, we promise to work hard at it. This rush of adrenaline gives us new hope and energy, and we are pumped and ready to take on the challenge of learning new things. Soon, however, our daily chores and routines begin to set in and seem to work against us. This is especially true for part-time or mature students who need to go to work and, in some cases, raise a family.

Before long we find ourselves running behind and unable to catch up. We do not have enough hours in the day to complete everything we need to do. Three weeks into the course, we begin to think about giving up and repeating the course in the next semester, which is a costly proposition. But the fact remains that all of us have twenty-four hours in a day. If others can do it, why can't we? But how did they do it? Do they have a secret recipe for successfully passing the exam? These are very good questions. Let us now try to analyze and crack the first secret of success.

The secret is to maintain the momentum after signing up for a course and then continuing on a disciplined approach to study until the final exam. There is no magic pill or medicine. You need to work hard for it. To do that, you need to have a good study plan.

The first week after signing up for a course of study is a crucial time of planning and seeing the big picture. You need a good study plan to daily guide your efforts. Your parents or teachers have probably told you that every successful event starts with a good plan, and a good plan breeds success. This is true.

What makes a good study plan? I am sure that planning is not new to you. You probably have executed hundreds of plans. Some of them just sit in your head, like planning to go swimming on a weekend. You simply do it as a matter of fact, as you have done it many times before. Also, you are not particularly concerned about the outcome or result. If the swimming pool is closed when you arrived, it is not the end of the world. You just go home and return the next day.

Some events require a little more planning, as failure to do so may cost a lot of time and money. Going on a ski trip 500 kilometres away from home requires careful planning, likely weeks in advance. The plan will include taking time off work, booking the ski hill and hotel room, paying for the ski pass, and other details. You need to write down all the pertinent information on a piece of paper and also mark the calendar. Failure to plan carefully for the trip could result in a significant financial loss to you and turn a happy vacation into an event you would rather forget.

I hope you now get the idea. A good study plan must be comprehensive, full of details, cater to important life events, and contain sufficient flexibility for you to respond to unexpected events. Study plans can cover several months or even years; however, our focus is on passing a course of study, so we will focus on a three to four month period.

To develop a good study plan, you will need to complete all of the following within the first week after registering for the course:

- Collect all the study materials and bring them home as soon as possible.

- Purchase or obtain a blank calendar, one in which you can write in the empty square for each day (see appendix). Better still, use Outlook calendar on the computer.

- Glance over the entire course materials from the beginning to the end several times.

- Find out how many chapters are covered and how they are organized.

- Jot down the theme of each chapter, its course objective, and what you are supposed to have learned after completing it.

- Browse through the assignments in each chapter and determine the deadlines for each submission.

- Take out the blank calendar and start marking down the deadline for the submission for each assignment and the date for each test (quiz, interim exam, final exam, etc.).

- On the same calendar, mark down the important personal events of your life, such as the birthdays of your loved ones, anniversary dates, vacation days, etc.

THE 7-11 METHOD

- If you are working, mark down the important events of your work life, such as the deadlines for month-end processing, important sales events and functions, projects deadlines, etc.

By this time your blank calendar is looking rather full. In fact, you will most likely be running out of space in each little square. Getting a bigger calendar will definitely help. I have been using the A4 size paper (8.5" by 11") for each calendar month, and that works well. You can also use the electronic calendar on your computer to achieve the same results.

Filling out the calendar gives you a bird's eye view of the entire course and how it will impact your daily life as you start the studying process. We all have a life to live, and studying for a course should not consume us to the point of giving up the important things or events that matter. After all, we are not entirely doing the course just for ourselves. We are also doing it for our loved ones. We want them to know that even though we have taken up the course of study, we care enough to include them in the process, as we need their ongoing support. In other words, this is not a lone ranger, one-person journey, but rather a collective journey of a united family with a common goal of ensuring that you will be successful in completing the course of study.

I have provided an example of what a good study plan looks like by completing a detailed, month-by-month calendar in the appendices at the end of the manual. I have used this approach for all of my courses over many years, and it has never failed me. I can confidently say that if you follow this approach, you will experience success. I recommend that you start by using the blank calendar provided in the Appendix or use the Outlook calendar on the computer to start crafting your own study plan.

Please remember that changes may have to be made and more life events added as you progress in your studies. This is normal; however, what cannot be changed is the deadline for each assignment and the exam date. They have been set by the professional bodies organizing the exam and will not change—unless there is a natural disaster in your area!

Maintaining a systematic and disciplined approach to studying is crucial once the course starts. It becomes increasingly important as you approach the final month of study and the last week and day before the final exam. We will discuss more about this in the next few chapters.

Chapter 3
First Month After The Course Starts

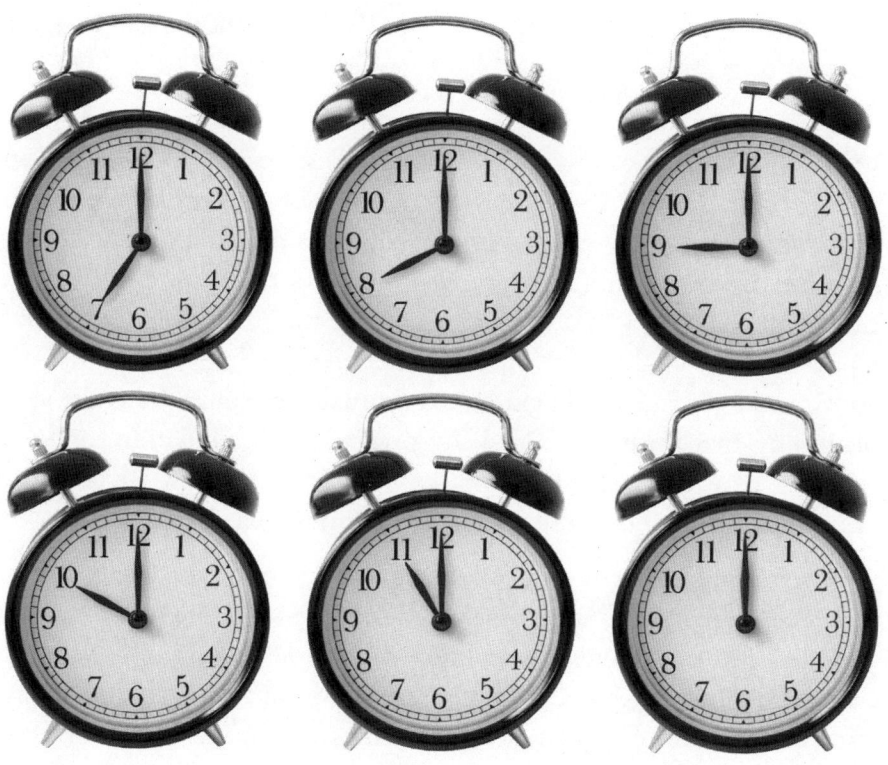

By now you should have gotten into the routine of studying; however, many students will still be trying to adjust to the new reality of keeping up with the "normal" daily life and finding time to cope with the humungous task of taking on a new course. Changes to our daily routine are never easy and always present a challenge. Unfortunately, there aren't many options to choose from other than adjusting your priorities to ensure that you will pass the required exams.

There are many types of students. The three most common ones are full-time students, part-time students who work odd jobs, and part-time students with careers and working regular 9 to 5 jobs (who may also be raising a family). Some may experience all three over the course of their studies. Full-time students are the luckiest as they only have to worry about school. Part-time student working odd jobs have additional flexibility, as more time is available for study when they are not working.

A person with a career working a regular job, or a married student with a spouse and possibly kid/s, has many responsibilities to juggle on a daily basis. This is no easy task. The constant pressure of life sometime means that you are living on the edge of a cliff and could fall over anytime. I belonged to the third category, and believe me, it was not easy. I prayed a lot and always reminded myself that all I needed was a pass so that I could move on to the next course. I also knew that if I continued to pass, I would graduate eventually. I realized from the very beginning that once I obtained my professional designation, nobody would ever ask me about my marks in specific courses. I had many borderline passes, but I also aced many subjects that I am good at.

After studying for several weeks into the course, you should have developed a regular routine that you adhere to until the final exam. If you are a full-time student, you know what time you need to wake up in the morning to get ready for classes. You have a timetable and plan your calendar carefully, attend the lectures during the day, complete the assignments on the same afternoon, and have plenty of time to relax and enjoy yourself in the evening and over the weekend. It is important that you pre-read all course materials before showing up for classes. That way you will be able to connect better and understand where the key points are when listening to the lecturer. You will also be able to answer the assignment questions better, allowing you to ace the course. As a full-time student, I would suggest that you always aim to ace the exam. You should try to achieve your best and give 100 per cent. That way, if you fall short for whatever reason, you will still be able to pass and move on.

If you are studying part-time because you need to go to work or raise a family, you really only have the evenings or weekends to study for the course. If you need to attend classes during the week, this will further cut down on the amount of personal time you have available to concentrate on your course. To address this challenge, I have developed the 7-11 formula. I have used this formula to achieve my successes, and I believe you can do it too. This formula should be used every day throughout the course until the final exam day.

The 7-11 formula involves devoting four-hour blocks of study time to the course. If you work a regular 9 to 5 job, you will devote the hours from 7:00 p.m. to 11:00 p.m. You will either be attending the class, working on your assignments, or studying the course materials. Over the weekend, the four-hour block of study time will run from 7:00 a.m. to 11:00 a.m. and then from 7:00 p.m. to 11:00 p.m. The rest of the hours will be your free time to spend however you want.

You may ask, "Why 7-11". Most professional accountancy exams are conducted in the evening, starting at 6.00 or 7.00 and usually lasting for three to four hours. During this time you must be at your best both physically and mentally in order to do well on the exam. This will not happen by accident. You need to train yourself for it. In other words, you need to accustom your body and your brain to function at peak performance during these hours of the day/night. Sticking to these hours throughout the duration of your course leading up to the final exam day is the best way to go. You will likely feel exhausted during the first few weeks, but it will get better and you will eventually get used to it after the first month.

If you are like me with a full-time, demanding job and a family, extra effort will be required in order to finish the course successfully. As a family person, your main goal should be to pass the course. Let's face it ... acing it will be a bonus. You will face many unexpected events and challenges, as you have a family to look after. Hours will be lost

THE 7-11 METHOD

within the 7-11 timeframe and will have to be made up, so you will need to improvise and adapt to the 7-11+ formula.

The + sign in the 7-11 formula means one to two more hours of studying time for each block—in other words, from 7:00 p.m. to midnight or 1:00 a.m. during the week. On the weekend, it will be from 7:00 a.m. to noon or 1:00 p.m., along with the same hours in the evening as on the weekdays. This is a grueling schedule to say the least, entailing massive sacrifices for the family. In order to ensure that the family is not neglected, I strongly recommend that you skip Friday night and all of Saturday to devote to your family. The amount of time you give up will be compensated by the additional hours you put in from Sunday to Thursday. Remember my advice: As a family person, your main objective is to pass the exam, and acing it will be a bonus. After all, what is the point of achieving a distinction in your studies but neglecting your precious family and possibly losing your marriage or kids?

The following is a summary of the 7-11 and 7-11+ formula:

- 7-11 means devoting the hours of 7:00 to 11:00 in the evening to studying during the week, and from 7:00 a.m. to 11:00 a.m. and 7:00 p.m. to 11:00 p.m. on weekends.
- 7-11+ means devoting the hours of 7:00 p.m. to 12:00 a.m. or 1:00 a.m. to studying during the week, and 7:00 a.m. to 12:00 p.m. or 1:00 p.m. and 7:00 p.m. to 12:00 a.m. or 1:00 a.m. on weekends.

Following a disciplined routine during the first month of the course will ensure that you are on the right path to success. This is a crucial time, and from my own personal experience, the urge to give up is also strongest during this month. You need to constantly remind yourself that you can do it. Following the above suggested schedule is not easy, but if you can adhere to it 80 per cent of the time, you should be able to pass the course quite comfortably ... provided you also follow the advice given in the next few chapters.

Chapter 4
Subsequent Months

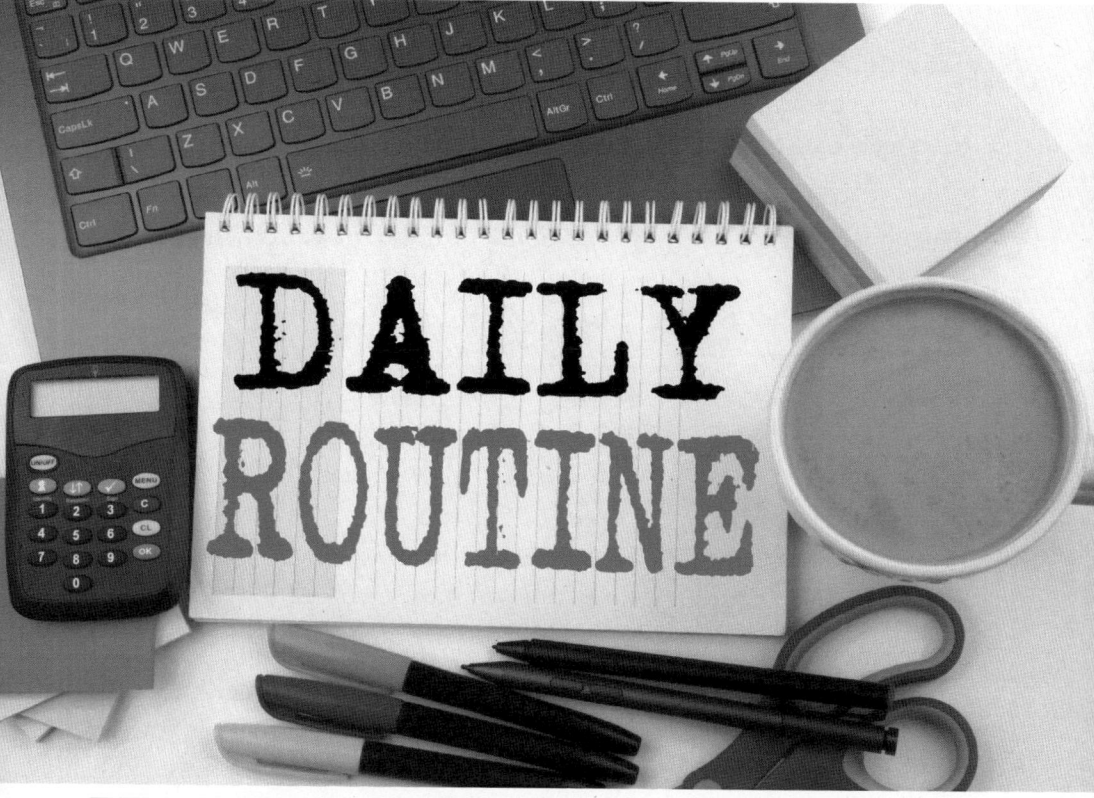

To be successful in anything, developing a disciplined routine plays an important role. Studying for a course and passing exams is no different. As a full-time student, the routine of going to school, which is what everyone does from a very young age, should not present any difficulties or challenges. It becomes your second nature. You just do it. However, as you grow older and join the workforce, many life events come at you and it is necessary to re-learn the skills of how to study and write exam. Studying for a professional exam does require additional commitments, but it will also bring you success in your career.

Professional study requires the individual to acquire work experience while learning new academic knowledge. It is believed that studying while working is more effective for professionals because they have opportunities to apply what they are learning to the real world at work. Studying part-time alone, or raising a family while working a full-time job, has become the norm, and many professional accountants can testify to it. The big accounting firms recruit the brightest graduates from university and encourage them to pursue professional accountancy designation while working for the firm.

Every student has other responsibilities and commitments other than studying that must be met. Some of these may affect the student emotionally, such as taking care of a sick family member. These responsibilities must not be neglected or ignored throughout the study plan. It is equally important to spend sufficient time attending to important family events or special requests at work. Meeting the needs of family members and ensuring harmony at the workplace is as important as spending time studying. Going into the exam hall feeling emotionally unstable or unable to concentrate either due to unresolved family issues or an adverse workplace event can mean the difference between a pass or fail, regardless of how well you have prepared for the exam.

In summary, developing a routine you are comfortable with and adhering to it as much as you can during the subsequent months leading up to the final exam day is the key to success, whether you are a full-time student, studying part-time alone, or raising a family while working a full-time job. Just like competing in the Olympics, your ability to win a medal can be easily lost if you are struggling emotionally, despite how hard work or how many hours or years you put into training for the event.

The following dos and don'ts serve as a good reminder as you immerse yourself in your studies while preparing for the exam during the subsequent months leading up to the final exam day:

- Do take time off frequently to unwind and relax to reflect on your study, your work, and your loved ones.
- Do remain focused on your goal of passing the exam.
- Do remember that the course you are studying is not the be all and end all.
- Do remember to celebrate major events in your and your family's life during the study period, even if they occur on the day before the final exam.
- Do feel confident that you have prepared well and that passing the final exam is not an issue.
- Do try to make up for lost time due to unexpected events that impact your study plan.
- Do avoid alcohol, drugs, or any stimulants that may affect your emotional or mental state or your physical health during the study period, especially during the last few days before the final exam.
- Don't let minor distractions or setbacks affect your study plan.
- Don't let your emotions affect your concentration while you study.
- Don't worry about what other students may have done in their study time. It is what you are doing to prepare for the exam that matters.
- Don't give up once you start the course. Stay focused and keep moving forward.
- Don't worry if you find it difficult to understand certain chapters of the course, or if you miss a few classes. Your goal is not to score 100 per cent but to simply pass the exam.
- Don't ever try to cheat during the final exam, because once you are caught, it will mean the end of your professional career even before you start.

Chapter 5
One Month Before The Final Exam

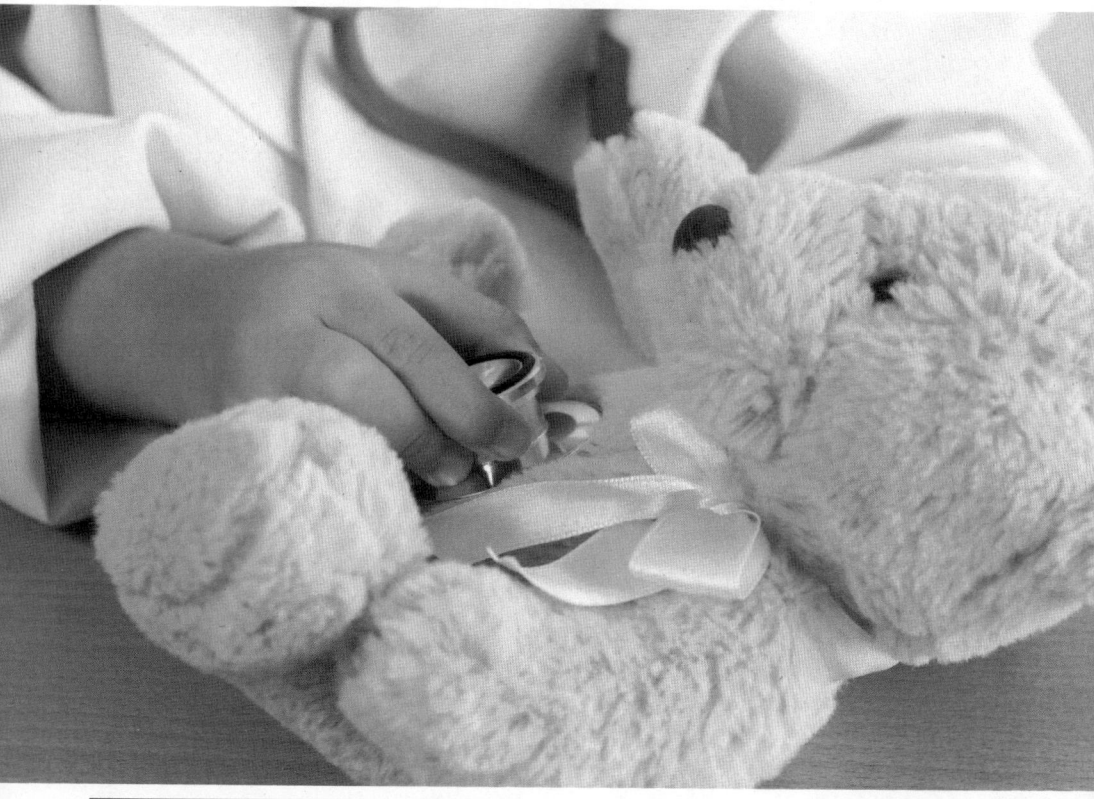

The month leading up to the final exam day is the most important period of the entire study plan. By now you should have covered more than 75 per cent of your course material, and you can almost see the light at the end of the tunnel. If you have been a disciplined student, you are quite happy that you are almost done with the course, and you are looking forward to finishing it so that you can move on to another course or go on that well-deserved vacation.

Unfortunately, many students will be playing catch-up either on their reading or completing the required assignments. Panic may start creeping in, and the desire to give up may form again out of fear of failing the exam. If you can get your money back, this is the time to throw in the towel and call it quits; however, most course fees are not refundable. Losing your money and all the earlier effort is simply not worth it. This situation is not uncommon, as procrastination is in the blood of many students. You need to bite the bullet and soldier on until you reach the finish line. Remember, you do not need to score 100 per cent to pass the exam.

This is also the time to consider writing a mock exam. Mock exams are like real exams, conducted on the same day and time as when the real thing will take place. In other words, if your exam is on a Wednesday night starting at 7.00 and ending at 10.00, then you will write the mock exam on the same day and time. I highly recommend that you write at least two mock exams during the month leading up to the final exam. This may seem like a silly proposal; however, you will be amazed at how much confidence you gain from these practice runs. All successful events in the world, including the Olympic opening and closing ceremonies, are rehearsed to ensure that when the actual events unfold, they will be spectacular and near-perfect.

To write the mock exam, you need to obtain past years' exam papers, which can usually be purchased from the same company that supplies your study materials, or from senior students who have completed the course. Most of them come with model answers as well. After each mock exam, carefully compare your answers with the model answers to ensure that you are "on the money" with what is required.

You need to purchase at least five years' worth of past questions and answers (Q&A). I normally order up to ten years if they are available. It is worth every penny! You will be surprised to learn that most of the questions are simply a variation of the same topic. I have personally seen some exam papers ask exactly the same questions year after year, with the same model answers. This is where you hit the jackpot and can expect full marks if you put down the answer the examiner wants. You will also be able to quickly finish the question (probably in less than half of the time allotted) and move on to the next one.

The following are some of the important tasks you need to perform at this important milestone of your study plan:

- Take stock of what you have completed to date and make plans to catch-up on what is lacking.

- Review your calendar carefully to ensure that you will be able to finish your studying and write the final exam on the day assigned. In other words, reschedule any upcoming appointments or events that may conflict with your exam.

- Start reviewing all assignments, including past years' exams, to ensure that you have understood the course materials thoroughly and are able to answer exam questions.

- Start writing mock exams on the day and hour the actual exam will be conducted. This will give you a feel of the real thing. Repeat this at least two times leading up to the actual exam day.

As you are working your way through the month and inching closer to the final exam, you will need to build up the momentum. When you hit the middle of the last month, you will be less than two weeks away from the final exam. Most classes should also come to an end, and you usually will have about two weeks left to prepare for the exam. These last two weeks are even more crucial than the others, and we will discuss them in the next chapter.

Chapter 6
Two Weeks Before The Final Exam

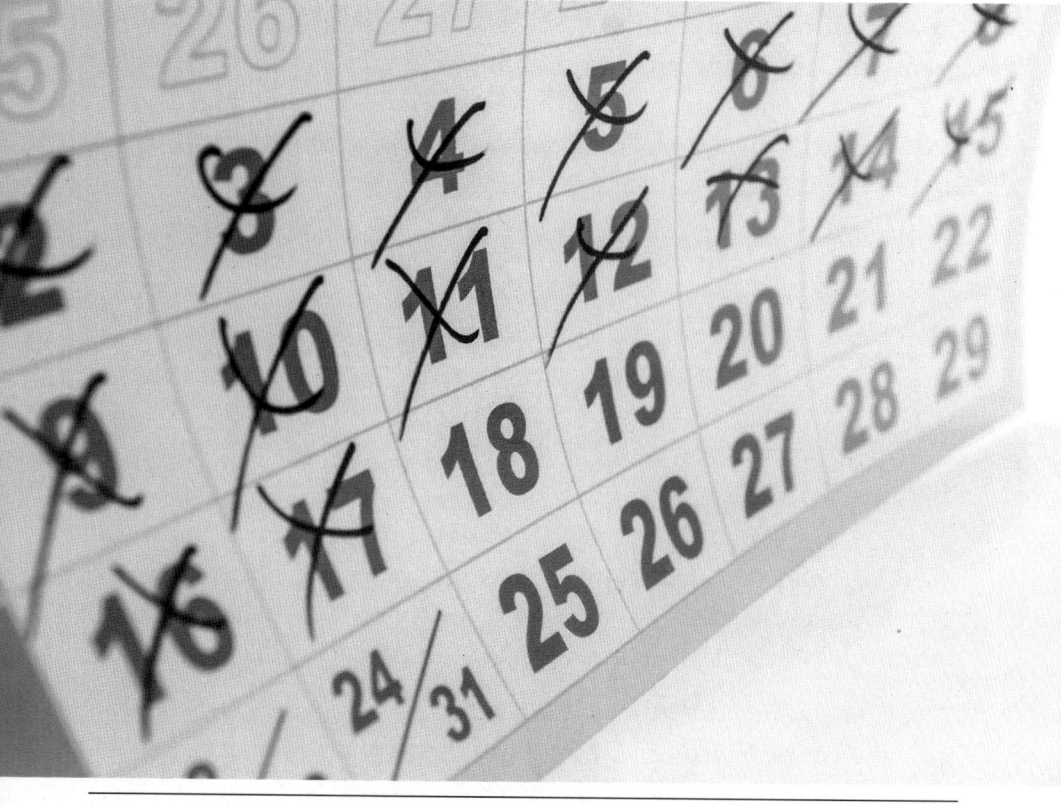

Two weeks before the final exam, the regular class usually ends and students get ready for the final exam. By now you should have completed your reading materials, including getting through all your assignments to qualify to sit for the final exam. Many students, however, feel apprehensive because the last few chapters of the course often present some challenges. If you are unsure about what you have learned in those chapters, do not let it overly bother you. It may only represent 10 to 15 per cent of the whole exam and should not affect your chances of passing.

Most students will find out if they are eligible to write the final exam based on the average mark they have obtained on the submitted assignments. If you are short a few percentage points, you need to immediately appeal to your course instructor and provide a good reason as to why you should be allowed to write the final exam. All course instructors are human too, and permission to write the final exam will usually be granted on compassionate grounds. However, don't stretch your luck too far by giving ridiculous or unbelievable reasons, such as "my pet lizard died" or "I was paralyzed for several days and was unable to complete the assignment."

The last two weeks before the exam is a time for review and revision. It is not the time to learn new concepts or cover new materials. This is the time when you need to be able to answer "most" of the questions from the materials covered in the course, whether from the first chapter or the last chapter. I use the word "most" because nobody knows what the actual exam questions will look like. As long as you know the overall concept of the course material, that should be sufficient.

A strategic use of each hour of each day during these last two weeks is critical, and you need to plan carefully on an hour by hour basis. This is where the countdown begins. The following is what you need to consider doing in the last twelve days leading up to the final exam:

- Day 12—review at least 10 per cent of all materials covered in the course, starting with the first chapter and browsing through each chapter and the assignments completed. Review the answers to past years' Q&As on similar topics. Read out loud or in your head the objectives and major concepts covered and how you will answer the questions presented. Memorizing the main points covered will help.

- Day 11—review the next 10 per cent of all materials covered in the course and repeat the same procedures as on Day 12.

- Day 10—review the next 10 per cent of all materials covered in the course and repeat the same procedures as on Day 12.
- Day 9—review the next 10 per cent of all materials covered in the course and repeat the same procedures as on Day 12.
- Day 8—review the next 10 per cent of all materials covered in the course and repeat the same procedures as on Day 12.
- Day 7—review the next 10 per cent of all materials covered in the course and repeat the same procedures as on Day 12.
- Day 6—review the next 10 per cent of all materials covered in the course and repeat the same procedures as on Day 12.
- Day 5—review the next 10 per cent of all materials covered in the course and repeat the same procedures as on Day 12.
- Day 4—review the next 10 per cent of all materials covered in the course and repeat the same procedures as on Day 12.
- Day 3—review the next 10 per cent of all materials covered in the course and repeat the same procedures as on Day 12.

You have now revised or covered 100 per cent of the course materials in ten days and you should feel pretty confident that you have a good grasp of each lesson. At this stage, passing the exam is quite certain, so the two remaining days focus on how you may ace the exam.

- Day 2—You are now just forty-eight hours away from your final exam day. Sit back and browse through all the course materials today. Keep telling yourself that you have been working hard and are looking forward to laying it all out in the exam hall to show that you really know the stuff you have been studying. However, remember that you are not there yet and should not let overconfidence set in and overtake you.

I would normally take it really easy on the last two days before the big final exam. If you like sports, going out for a jog or swim in the evening will help you to relax more. Some students will try to jam everything into the last two days, even burning the midnight oil to

THE 7-11 METHOD

study because they are not following the advice given so far and are not well prepared for the exam. But remember ... this is not you. You have done your best and should feel confident about it. Don't try to recall every topic in your head or panic if you can't remember everything. Nobody can, and this is normal. If you have prepared well, the important facts will come to you naturally when you are sitting in the examination hall answering the questions.

Chapter 7
The Day Before The Final Exam

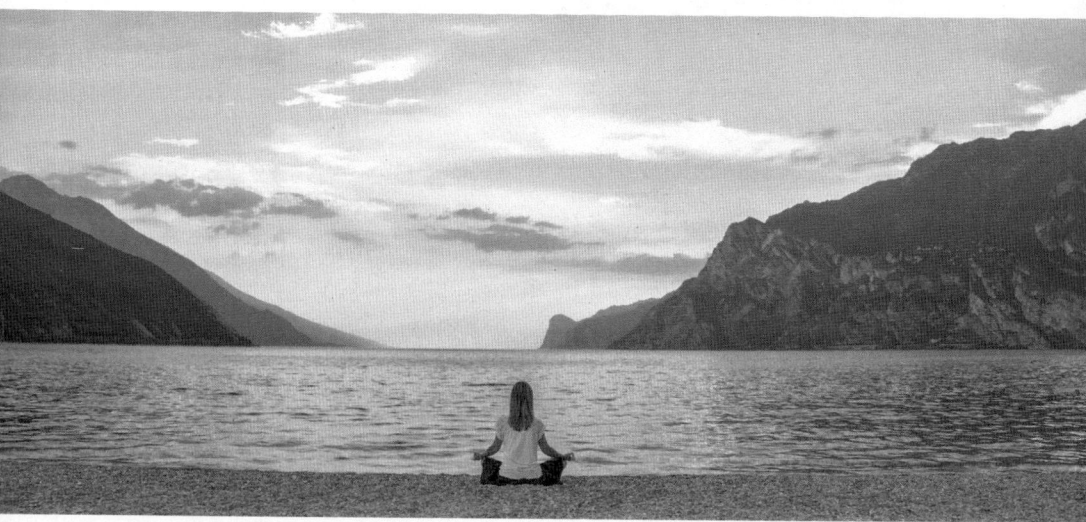

The last day before the final exam should be a calm day. You are almost there! You feel ready and can't wait for tomorrow to arrive. Good luck to you! However, this can be a nerve-racking day if you are a student like me, where you are just about 60 per cent sure of what you have learned so far. You have not finished the last two chapters of the course. Your boss in the office requires that you must complete the project today or else you may be fired. At home, your spouse, girlfriend, or boyfriend, although sympathetic to you all along, suddenly appears to be on the verge of blowing her/his top over all the suffering and chores you have bestowed on them over the last several months. The kids are not cooperating either, and you feel like taping their mounts, hands, and legs with duct tape so that you can have some peace and quiet at home to get ready for the exam tomorrow.

THE 7-11 METHOD

No matter how well you have prepared for the exam, the day before the exam is definitely not the day you should feel regret about what could have been done, or worry about what else you need to study. This is the day when you need to take a deep breath and reflect on all the hard work you have put in getting ready for the BIG day tomorrow. This is it, and there is no other way or turning back. Tomorrow will come whether you are ready or not.

Below are some of the activities I would strongly recommend you do today. They have worked for me all these years, and I am sure you will find some of them very useful.

- If you can, take the day off from work and wake up at 6:00 a.m. After a hearty breakfast, go to your usual study area and pull out the summary notes you have prepared for each chapter of the course. Begin reviewing the materials and continue for several hours until you finish all of them.
- Try to read the materials out loud while doodling key words and major concepts on a piece of paper.
- Complete the above before noon and after that eat a healthy lunch.
- Return from lunch and repeat the process above until you are done, hopefully before dinner time at 6:00 p.m. This is where you stop. Walk away from your study area and go find a place where you can relax. Do not return to your study area again until the final exam is over.
- Go to bed early tonight, preferably before 10:00 p.m. I strongly recommend against burning the midnight oil and trying to catch-up on the last few pages of the notes, regardless of your preparedness, because you need all the rest you can get to recharge your body for the important day tomorrow.

Unfortunately, some students will do exactly the opposite and study into the wee hours of the night and early morning. This will do more harm than good, because even though your mind is willing, your body will not be able to take it. As a result, you will feel tired tomorrow and will not be in your top form when the time comes to sit in the exam hall. Both your mind and body need to rest adequately for the night in order to write a successful exam; therefore, you need to avoid the temptation of burning the midnight oil. It is simply not worth it.

Chapter 8
The Final Exam Day

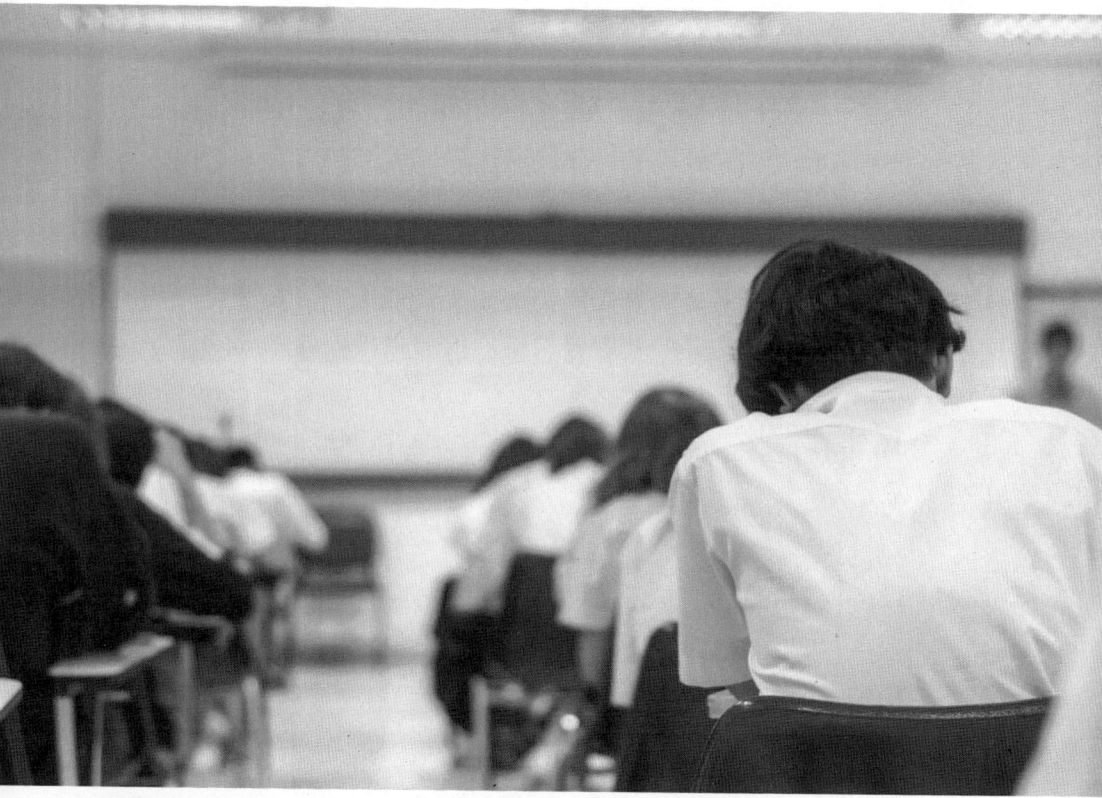

The final exam day is the day you have been preparing for over the last several months. You should take the day off from work and prepare for the hour that will soon arrive. This can be a day of reckoning, so feeling anxious throughout the day is normal. This is what you have been waiting for. You should feel really good about yourself today. You know you have prepared well for it. Think positively throughout the day and keep reminding yourself that you can do it. You have studied hard enough, practiced enough, and can't wait to put all your hard work to good use in the exam hall today/tonight. There is really nothing much to do other than feel confident that you are going to make it. Carry the positive energy with you throughout the day and feel happy about it.

Do not book any other major event for today. You should also avoid strenuous exercise, partying, or drinking until the exam is over. Avoid any heavy-duty activities. You need to feel calm and relaxed throughout the day. For those who do not feel quite ready for the exam, this can be a day when your migraine may start acting up. You may feel moody and even angry. My advice is to realize that it may be too late to feel sorry about it, so you simply need to accept the fact and be ready for the exam regardless. Finding a quiet place to be left alone will usually help. Listening to soft melodies or your favourite music may improve your mood. Do not give up easily, as passing the exam does not require you to score 100 per cent. You may be able to scrape through the exam and pass it.

The following is the TO DO list for the day:

- Arrive at the exam centre at least an hour before the exam start time.

- Bring with you your favourite music and listen to it while waiting to enter the exam hall.

- You will notice that many students are busy reading their notes and feeling very nervous. Do not be intimidated by what you see, because you are not one of them. You are well prepared for the exam, and they are not.

- Thirty minutes before the exam starts, go to the washroom, wash your hands, and look into the mirror and said "I am ready."

- Walk into the exam hall confidently and find your spot if the seat is assigned; otherwise, always sit at the front to avoid being distracted by other students during the exam.

- Take out your writing materials and place your watch on the corner of the desk so that you can look at it easily.
- Before the exam paper is distributed, make sure that you write down your name or assigned exam candidate number on the answer sheet correctly and on each sheet of the answer paper.
- Once the exam paper is distributed, wait for the instructions to begin. Take a deep breath, relax, and be ready.
- Once the exam proctor says you can start, spend the first five minutes doing the following:
    - Look at the front cover of the exam paper to make sure you received the right exam paper.
    - Quickly flip through the entire exam paper and glance through all the questions.
    - Look for any questions that you are most familiar with and number them in the order you want to answer them.
    - Divide the amount of time to be spent on each question based on the marks allotted and write that down beside the question number.
- Start answering the questions you are most familiar with first and progress from there.
- Keep a close eye on the watch to ensure that you do not exceed the time allotted for each question.
- If you find a particular question especially difficult, do not panic, because other students will probably find it hard too. Leave this to the last and then try your best to complete answering the question at the end.

THE 7-11 METHOD

Extremely Important: You MUST try to answer ALL questions on the exam paper.

- If you find yourself in the enviable position of finishing all the questions before the time is up, DO NOT LEAVE THE EXAM HALL EARLY. Use the additional time to check through all the answers and perfect each one of them as much as you can. This is the difference between simply passing an exam and acing it. Remember, you have paid for the time to sit for this exam, so make the best of every minute of it.

- Once you have completed answering all the questions, number your answer sheets numerically. If you used twenty sheets of paper, then number each sheet in the order of 1/20, 2/20 ... 20/20. This will ensure that all the answer sheets are complete before you hand them in.

- Once the answer sheets are collected by the exam proctor, your task is complete. Collect your writing materials and leave the exam hall.

Finish writing an exam is an achievement in itself, as you have spent countless hours preparing for it. You should feel good and proud regardless of how well you have performed. I usually walk away from the exam hall and find a quiet place to shout out loud, "I did it!" It also doesn't hurt to visit the washroom again so that you have a comfortable ride home.

Chapter 9
The Day After

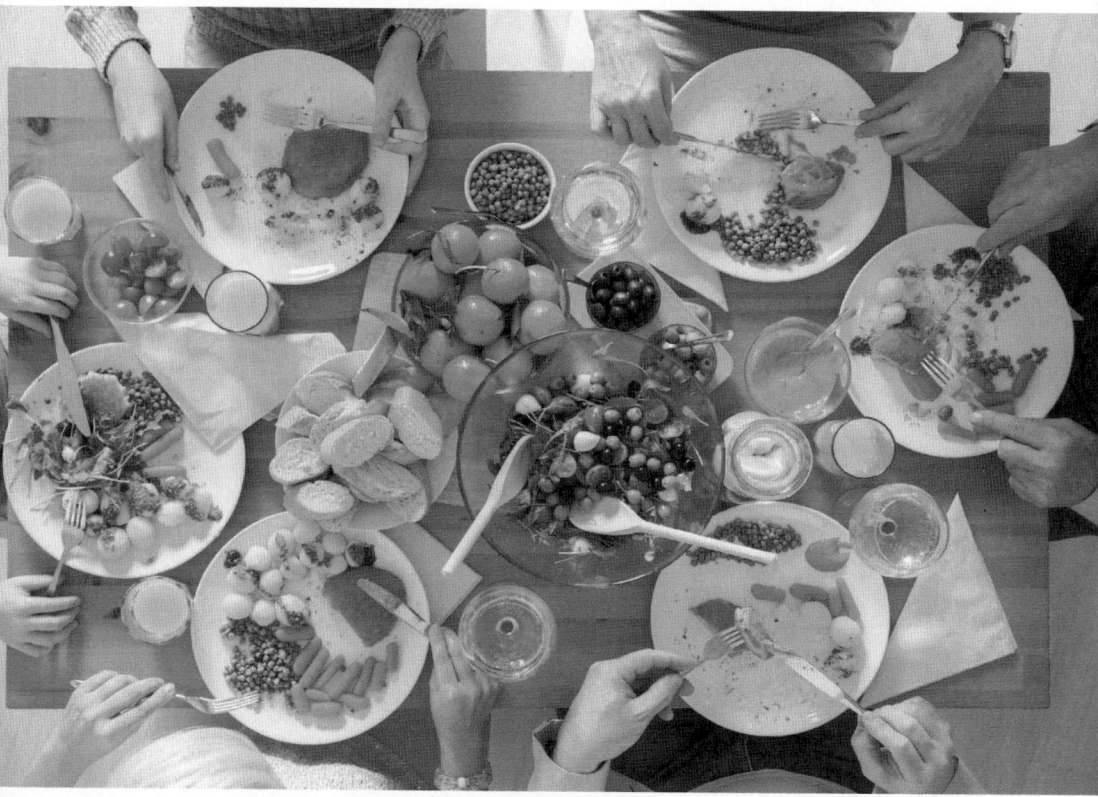

The day after the final exam is no ordinary day for many students. Regardless of how well you might feel you did on the exam, you deserve a break and should take it easy, relax, and enjoy the day off from studying. If you have a family, this is also the day you should kiss your loved ones and take them out for a good meal for supporting you all along.

You may want to assess your chances of success in passing the exam. I would recommend that you try to recall all the exam questions by writing them down on a piece of paper, since usually you can't take the exam booklet out of the exam hall. They are collected and returned to the examination body after each exam. Once the questions are written down, you can check your notes over the next several days to determine if you answered all the questions correctly. This way you should be able to determine your chances of passing the exam. It is never too early to start preparing the study plan for the next course if you are pretty sure that you are going to make it.

People often ask what they should do with all the notes they prepared for the exams. You can certainly recycle the papers and give away or sell the books. I usually keep mine for several years until I complete all the courses and graduate. If any future courses are related to past ones, I may not need to re-write the notes.

I would advise that you not give your notes, especially those related to assignments, to other students studying the same course. This is to avoid the accusation of being an accessory to plagiarism in the event that your work is copied or used inappropriately. As a professional, your integrity and reputation is paramount. Once you are accused of any wrongdoing, it is difficult to clear your good name. Trying to be helpful may cause you unnecessary grief in the end.

In closing, I truly hope that this book has provided you with some practical advice that you can use to prepare for and pass your exams. I wish you Godspeed in becoming a true professional in the not-too-distant future.

Appendix A1
Sample Planning Calendar
(After The Course Registration)

MONTH: JANUARY

Monday	Tuesday	Wednesday	Thursday	Friday	Saturday	Sunday
1 Course registered and feeling good and motivated Inform family members and office colleagues & superior in office Start thinking about the study strategy Take out blank planning calendar	2 Review entire course materials Determine chapters to cover Glance through chapter objective Glance through assignments to complete and identify deadlines Identify important life events	3 Continue reviewing course materials Decide how to capture important ideas and concepts into Summary Notes Continue to identify important life events, deadlines, etc.	4 Repeat Day 2 & 3 activities Mum's birthday – dinner at 6.30 p.m.	5 Repeat Day 2 & 3 activities	6 Repeat Day 2 & 3 activities Complete filling of calendars for all course activities & important life events Attend concert	7 Repeat Day 2 & 3 activities Get ready to start class next week Pre-read Chapter 1 materials
8 **Start Chapter 1** Read Chapter 1 materials Start reviewing assignment questions Department staff meeting	9 **Attend evening class from 6:00 to 9.00** Revise materials covered in class Continue reviewing assignment questions	10 Complete reading / reviewing chapter materials Start answering assignment questions **Buy flowers**	11 **Attend evening class from 6:00 to 9.00** Review materials covered in class Continue answering assignment questions	12 Revise course materials and continue answering assignment questions **Movie at 8.00 p.m.**	13 Complete answering all assignment questions & submit Prepare Summary Notes for materials covered **Family gathering**	14 Get ready to start class next week Pre-read Chapter 2 materials **Hockey night**

38

15	16	17	18	19	20	21
Start Chapter 2 Read Chapter 2 materials Start review assignment questions **Project A starts**	**Attend evening class from 6:00 to 9.00** Revise materials covered in class Continue reviewing assignment questions	Complete reading / reviewing chapter materials Start answering assignment questions **Budget meeting**	**Attend evening class from 6:00 to 9.00** Review materials covered in class Continue answering assignment questions	Revise course materials and continue answering assignment questions **Pub night with friends**	Complete answering all assignment questions & submit Prepare Summary Notes for materials covered	Get ready to start class next week Pre-read Chapter 3 materials **Baby shower for Emily**
22	23	24	25	26	27	28
Start Chapter 3 Read Chapter 3 materials Start reviewing assignment questions **Doctor's appointment**	**Attend evening class from 6:00 to 9.00** Revise materials covered in class Continue reviewing assignment questions	Complete reading / reviewing chapter materials Start answering assignment questions **Month-end starts**	**Attend evening class from 6:00 to 9.00** Review materials covered in class Continue answering assignment questions	Revise course materials and continue answering assignment questions **Project A due today**	Complete answering all assignment questions & submit Prepare Summary Notes for materials covered	Get ready to start class next week Pre-read Chapter 4 materials **Hockey night**
29	30	31				
Start Chapter 4 Read Chapter 4 materials Start reviewing assignment questions	**Attend evening class from 6:00 to 9.00** Revise materials covered in class Continue reviewing assignment questions	Complete reading / reviewing chapter materials Start answering assignment questions **Jen's birthday**				

Appendix A2
Sample Planning Calendar
(Subsequent Month)

MONTH: FEBRUARY						
Monday	Tuesday	Wednesday	Thursday	Friday	Saturday	Sunday
			1 Attend evening class from 6pm to 9.00pm Review materials covered in class Continue answering assignment questions	2 Revise course materials and continue answering assignment questions **Farewell lunch for Steve**	3 Complete answering all assignment questions & submit Prepare Summary Notes for materials covered **Picnic at the lake**	4 Getting ready to start class next week Pre-read Chapter 5 materials
5 **Start Chapter 5** Read Chapter 5 materials Start reviewing assignment questions **Call aunt Lily**	6 Attend evening class from 6:00 to 9.00 Revise materials covered in class Continue reviewing assignment questions	7 Complete reading / reviewing Chapter materials Start answering assignment questions **PTA meeting**	8 Attend evening class from 6:00 to 9.00 Review materials covered in class Continue answering assignment questions **MID TERM EXAM**	9 Revise course materials and continue answering assignment questions **Movie Night**	10 Complete answering all assignment questions & submit Prepare Summary Notes for materials covered **Family gathering**	11 Get ready to start class next week Pre-read Chapter 6 materials **Hockey night**

12	13	14	15	16	17	18
Out of town business trip from 12 to 15 **Start Chapter 6** Read Chapter 6 materials Start reviewing assignment questions	Out of town business trip from 12 to 15 Skip evening class from 6:00 to 9.00 Continue reviewing assignment questions	Out of town business trip from 12 to 15 Complete reading / reviewing chapter materials Start answering assignment questions **Valentine Day**	Out of town business trip from 12 to 15 Skip evening class from 6:00 to 9.00 Continue answering assignment questions	Revise course materials and continue answering assignment questions **Pub night with friends**	Complete answering all assignment questions & submit Prepare Summary Notes for materials covered **Make up dinner for Valentine's Day**	Get ready to start class next week Pre-read Chapter 7 materials
19	20	21	22	23	24	25
Start Chapter 7 Read Chapter 7 materials Start reviewing assignment questions **Department staff meeting**	**Attend evening class from 6:00 to 9.00** Revise materials covered in class Continue reviewing assignment questions	Complete reading / reviewing chapter materials Start answering assignment questions **Month-end starts**	**Attend evening class from 6:00 to 9.00** Review materials covered in class Continue answering assignment questions	Revise course materials and continue answering assignment questions **Dentist's appointment**	Complete answering all assignment questions & submit Prepare Summary Notes for materials covered	Get ready to start class next week Pre-read Chapter 8 materials **Hockey night**
26	27	28				
Start Chapter 8 Read Chapter 8 materials Start reviewing assignment questions	**Attend evening class from 6:00 to 9.00** Revise materials covered in class Continue reviewing assignment questions	Complete reading / reviewing chapter materials Start answering assignment questions **Budget meeting**				

Appendix A3
Sample Planning Calendar
(One Month Before The Final Exam Day)

MONTH: MARCH

Monday	Tuesday	Wednesday	Thursday	Friday	Saturday	Sunday
			1 **One month to go** **Attend evening class from 6:00 to 9:00** Review materials covered in class Continue answering assignment questions	**2** Revise course materials and continue answering assignment questions **Friends coming over**	**3** Complete answering all assignment questions & submit Prepare Summary Notes for materials covered	**4** Get ready to start class next week Pre-read Chapter 9 materials **Dad's birthday – dinner at 6.30 p.m.**
5 **Start Chapter 9** Read Chapter 9 materials Start reviewing assignment questions **Submit expense report**	**6** **Attend evening class from 6:00 to 9:00** Revise materials covered in class Continue reviewing assignment questions	**7** **1st Mock Exam** Attempt past year exam at the same hour as the real Exam day Complete reading / reviewing chapter materials Start answering assignment questions	**8** **Attend evening class from 6:00 to 9:00** Review materials covered in class Continue answering assignment questions	**9** Revise course materials and continue answering assignment questions **Pickup uncle Joe at airport**	**10** Complete answering all assignment questions & submit Prepare Summary Notes for materials covered **Family gathering**	**11** Get ready to start class next week Pre-read Chapter 10 materials **Hockey night**
12 **Start Chapter 10** Read Chapter 10 materials	**13** **Attend evening class from 6:00 to 9:00** Revise materials covered in class	**14** **2nd Mock Exam** Attempt past year exam at the same hour as the real Exam day	**15** **Attend evening class from 6:00 to 9:00**	**16** **12 Days to go** Complete answering assignment questions	**17** **11 Days to go** Submit assignment online Prepare Summary Notes	**18** **10 Days to go** Review the NEXT 10% of the course work materials

Start reviewing assignment questions **Book spring break vacation**	Continue reviewing assignment questions	Complete reading / reviewing chapter materials Start answering assignment questions	Revise materials covered in class Continue answering assignment questions **Renew driver's licence**	Review the FIRST 10% of the course work materials Work through all assignments for related chapters Attempt related past years' Q/A	Review the NEXT 10% of the course work materials Work through all assignments for related chapters Attempt related past years' Q/A	Work through all assignments for related chapters Attempt related past years' Q/A **Anniversary dinner**
19 **9 Days to go** Review the NEXT 10% of the course work materials Work through all assignments for related chapters Attempt related past years' Q/A **Department staff meeting**	**20** **8 Days to go** Review the NEXT 10% of the course work materials Work through all assignments for related chapters Attempt related past years' Q/A	**21** **7 Days to go** Review the NEXT 10% of the course work materials Work through all assignments for related chapters Attempt related past years' Q/A **Month-end starts**	**22** **6 Days to go** Review the NEXT 10% of the course work materials Work through all assignments for related chapters Attempt related past years' Q/A **Budget meeting**	**23** **5 Days to go** Review the NEXT 10% of the course work materials Work through all assignments for related chapters Attempt related past years' Q/A **Pub night with friends**	**24** **4 Days to go** Review the NEXT 10% of the course work materials Work through all assignments for related chapters Attempt related past years' Q/A	**25** **3 Days to go** Review the LAST 10% of the course work materials Work through all assignments for related chapters Attempt related past years' Q/A **Note: 100% of course materials have now been reviewed**
26 **2 Days to go** Browse through all course materials again Review Summary Notes many times **Feeling confident and ready for the Exam**	**27** **1 Day to go** Take today and tomorrow off from work Review all Summary Notes **Go to bed by 10:00 p.m.**	**28** **FINAL EXAM DAY** Relax and no strenuous activities Quick review of Summary Notes **Arrive 1 Hour before exam starts**	**29** **The Day After** Take family out to celebrate **Start thinking about the next course** **Dinner at restaurant for 8**	**30**	**31**	

APPENDIX A4
Blank Planning Calendar

MONTH:						
Monday	Tuesday	Wednesday	Thursday	Friday	Saturday	Sunday
1	2	3	4	5	6	7
8	9	10	11	12	13	14

15	16	17	18	19	20	21
22	23	24	25	26	27	28
29	30	31				

Appendix B1
Sample Daily Timetable

Time	Monday	Tuesday	Wednesday	Thursday	Friday	Saturday	Sunday
6.00 a.m.	Wake Up	Wake Up	Wake Up	Wake Up	Wake Up	Wake Up	Wake Up
7.00 a.m.	Go to Work	Go to Work	Go to Work	Go to Work	Go to Work	Study	Study
8.00 a.m.	Office Hours	Office Hours	Office Hours	Office Hours	Office Hours	Study	Study
9.00 a.m.	Office Hours	Office Hours	Office Hours	Office Hours	Office Hours	Study	Study
10.00 a.m.	Office Hours	Office Hours	Office Hours	Office Hours	Office Hours	Study	Study
11.00 a.m.	Office Hours	Office Hours	Office Hours	Office Hours	Office Hours	Study	Study
12.00 p.m.	Lunch	Lunch	Lunch	Lunch	Lunch	Lunch	Lunch
1.00 p.m.	Office Hours	Office Hours	Office Hours	Office Hours	Office Hours	Personal	Family

	Monday	Tuesday	Wednesday	Thursday	Friday	Saturday	Sunday
2.00 p.m.	Office Hours	Office Hours	Office Hours	Office Hours	Office Hours	Personal	Family
3.00 p.m.	Office Hours	Office Hours	Office Hours	Office Hours	Office Hours	Personal	Family
4.00 p.m.	Office Hours	Office Hours	Office Hours	Office Hours	Office Hours	Personal	Family
5.00 p.m.	Dinner	Dinner	Dinner	Dinner	Dinner	Dinner	Dinner
6.00 p.m.	Family	Attend Class	Family	Attend Class	Family	Family	Family
7.00 p.m.	Study	Attend Class	Study	Attend Class	Family	Study	Study
8.00 p.m.	Study	Attend Class	Study	Attend Class	Family	Study	Study
9.00 p.m.	Study	Study	Study	Study	Family	Study	Study
10.00 p.m.	Study	Study	Study	Study	Family	Study	Study
11.00 p.m.	Study	Study	Study	Study	Family	Study	Study
12.00 a.m.	Go to Bed	Go to Bed	Go to Bed	Go to Bed	Go to Bed	Go to Bed	Go to Bed

APPENDIX B2
Blank Daily Timetable

Time	Monday	Tuesday	Wednesday	Thursday	Friday	Saturday	Sunday
6.00 a.m.							
7.00 a.m.							
8.00 a.m.							
9.00 a.m.							
10.00 a.m.							
11.00 a.m.							
12.00 p.m.							
1.00 p.m.							

2.00 p.m.	3.00 p.m.	4.00 p.m.	5.00 p.m.	6.00 p.m.	7.00 p.m.	8.00 p.m.	9.00 p.m.	10.00 p.m.	11.00 p.m.	12.00 a.m.

About the Author

Hin H. Leong, is a member in good standing of several prestigious professional accountancy bodies around the world including Canada, United Kingdom, Australia, Malaysia, and ASEAN. He sat and passed many exams while working at a full time job and raising a family, using the disciplined and systematic approach of the 7-11 method of study he developed that was perfected over time. He is now sharing his successful and proven method with you. Hin works as a Director of Audit for one of the world's largest natural resources company. He lives in Calgary, Alberta, Canada, home to the majestic Rocky Mountains, the pristine Lake Louise, the Calgary Flames professional ice hockey team, and the Calgary Stampeders professional football club.

Printed in Canada